YOUR KNOWLEDGE HAS VALUE

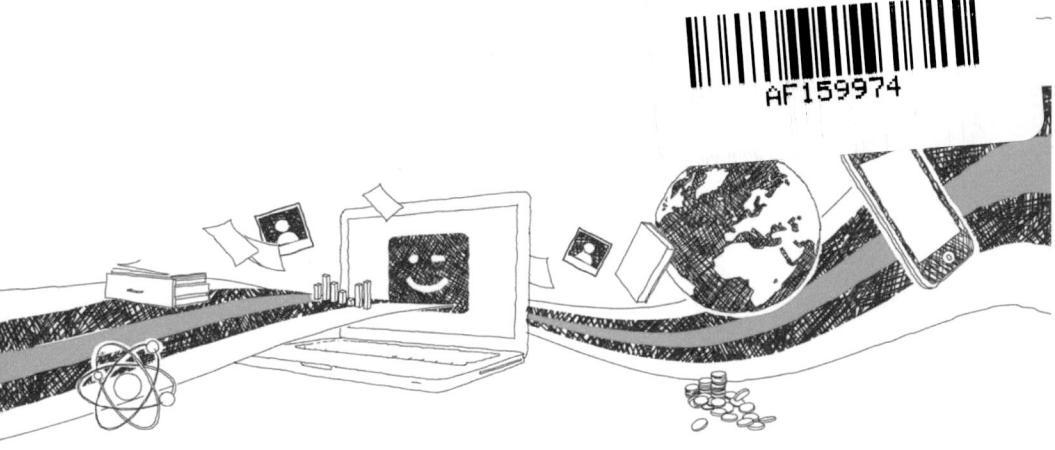

- We will publish your bachelor's and master's thesis, essays and papers

- Your own eBook and book - sold worldwide in all relevant shops

- Earn money with each sale

Upload your text at www.GRIN.com and publish for free

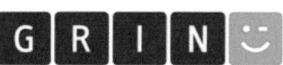

Bibliographic information published by the German National Library:

The German National Library lists this publication in the National Bibliography; detailed bibliographic data are available on the Internet at http://dnb.dnb.de .

This book is copyright material and must not be copied, reproduced, transferred, distributed, leased, licensed or publicly performed or used in any way except as specifically permitted in writing by the publishers, as allowed under the terms and conditions under which it was purchased or as strictly permitted by applicable copyright law. Any unauthorized distribution or use of this text may be a direct infringement of the author s and publisher s rights and those responsible may be liable in law accordingly.

Imprint:

Copyright © 2018 GRIN Verlag
Print and binding: Books on Demand GmbH, Norderstedt Germany
ISBN: 9783668630666

This book at GRIN:

https://www.grin.com/document/411948

Patrick Kimuyu

Hypercortisolism. Understanding "Cushing's Syndrome"

GRIN Verlag

GRIN - Your knowledge has value

Since its foundation in 1998, GRIN has specialized in publishing academic texts by students, college teachers and other academics as e-book and printed book. The website www.grin.com is an ideal platform for presenting term papers, final papers, scientific essays, dissertations and specialist books.

Visit us on the internet:

http://www.grin.com/

http://www.facebook.com/grincom

http://www.twitter.com/grin_com

Introduction

Hormones play integral biological roles in the body, primarily the regulation of body functions. Scientific research indicates that hormones regulate a range of body functions such as reproduction, metabolism, electrolyte balance, as well as, growth and development (Hiller-Sturmhöfel & Bartke, 1998). As such, the endocrine system is considered supreme in the regulation of biological processes of the body. Biologically, the endocrine system maintains effective communication among various body organs. This communication ensures homeostasis processes are maintained at constant levels, as well as, enabling the body to respond to changes in the external environment. From anatomical perspective, the endocrine system comprises of glands that are located at different regions of the body, which release hormones. The main components of the endocrine system are the hypothalamus, pituitary gland, thyroid gland, parathyroid gland, adrenal glands, pancreas, and the gonads. These glands release hormones through various regulatory hormonal cascades including the hypothalamic-pituitary-gonadal (HPG) axis, the hypothalamic-pituitary-adrenal (HPA) axis and the hypothalamic-pituitary-thyroidal (HPT) axis. As such, any disturbances in the regulatory hormonal cascades results into devastating medical conditions. For instance, disturbances in the HPA axis, primarily excessive release of adrenocorticotropic hormone (ACTH) results into Cushing's syndrome. Cushing's syndrome, also known as hypercortisolism is a disorder of the endocrine system that is characterized by excess release of cortisol. Cortisol plays various regulatory functions in all organs and tissues in the body; thus, Cushing's syndrome affects the entire body. Epidemiological data shows that Cushing's syndrome affects 10-15 per million people, annually (Newell-Price, Bertagna, Grossman & Nieman, 2006). Therefore, this research paper will provide a comprehensive overview of Cushing's syndrome. It will discuss the underlying pathology, symptoms, pathophysiology, diagnosis, and treatment of the disorder.

Pathology of Cushing's Syndrome

In retrospect, the pathology of the Cushing's syndrome is related to three main causes: overuse of anti-inflammatory drugs, excessive production of cortisol from adrenal tumors, or pituitary adenomas.

Iatrogenic Cushing's syndrome occurs develops due to the prolonged use of corticosteroids. In most cases, this is the common form of Cushing's syndrome that occurs among patients who are undergoing corticosteroid therapy for the treatment of chronic rheumatoid arthritis and asthma (Newell-Price et al., 2006). These medications are cortisol-based; thus, they increase the body's exposure to cortisol leading to the development of the Cushing's syndrome.

The second cause of Cushing's syndrome is pituitary tumors, commonly referred to as pituitary adenomas (Vassiliadil & Tsagarakis, 2007). Pituitary adenomas are usually are benign tumors that develop in the pituitary gland. These tumors increase the production of ACTH by the pituitary gland which, in turn, results into excessive production of cortisol in the body. Clinical literature refers to this condition as Cushing's disease, and it is the most common cause of Cushing's syndrome. According to epidemiological reports, pituitary adenomas account for an estimated 60-70% of all cases of Cushing's syndrome.

On the other hand, tumors in ACTH-producing tissues that are outside the pituitary gland can cause Cushing's syndrome. This condition is referred to as ectopic Cushing's syndrome (Vassiliadil & Tsagarakis, 2007). Examples of these malignant tumors include lung tumors, medullary carcinomas of the thyroid, pancreatic islet cell tumors, and thymomas. Of these tumors, lung tumors are the most common, accounting for more than 50% of all cases of ectopic Cushing's syndrome.

Excessive production of cortisol by adrenal tumors is the fourth cause of Cushing's syndrome (Vassiliadil & Tsagarakis, 2007). From a physiological perspective, adrenal adenomas, non-cancerous tumors, increases cortisol release from the adrenal gland into the bloodstream. Similarly, adrenocortical carcinomas increase the secretion of adrenal cortical hormones, primarily adrenal androgens and cortisol. It is apparent that adrenocortical carcinomas trigger a rapid onset of Cushing's syndrome due to their potential to produce high levels of cortisol.

Finally, inherited disorders of the endocrine glands, especially tumors are known to cause Cushing's syndrome, although this accounts for a few cases. This condition is referred to as familial Cushing's syndrome. There are two genetic conditions that are associated with familial Cushing's syndrome. The first predisposing genetic condition is known as multiple endocrine neoplasia type 1. This condition may lead to the development of hormone-secreting tumors in the pituitary gland, adrenal gland, pancreas, or parathyroid glands. The second condition is known as primary pigmented micronodular adrenal disease that affects young adults and children. This condition is characterized by the development of cortisol-secreting tumors in the adrenal glands, thus, the onset of symptoms of Cushing's syndrome.

Symptoms of Cushing's Syndrome

Clinically, Cushing's syndrome is characterized by its main symptoms. However, it is worth noting that its presentation exhibits demographic factors. This implies that symptoms vary from women to men, as well as children, although there are common symptoms. In most cases of Cushing's syndrome, a condition known as moon face in which the face appears round and red occurs. Another common symptom is weight gain which is caused by uneven accumulation of fat, primarily on the trunk (Hiller-Sturmhöfel & Bartke, 1998). People with Cushing's syndrome develop central obesity with fat accumulation in the chest, abdomen, the back of the neck, a condition known as the buffalo hump, and around the collar bone. In contrast, they show a characteristic fat loss from the buttocks, arms and legs.

Cushing's syndrome is also associated with skin changes. Most people with Cushing's syndrome exhibit thin skin that bruises easily (Hiller-Sturmhöfel & Bartke, 1998). Skin infections are also common among the patients. However, the appearance of a condition known as triae on the skin, especially on the thighs, abdomen and breasts serves as the main characteristic, exclusive with Cushing's syndrome. The purple mark ranges from half inch wide or more.

Similarly, Cushing's syndrome is characterized by muscle and bone changes. In reality, patients with Cushing's syndrome experience backache during routine activities (Hiller-Sturmhöfel & Bartke, 1998). They also experience episodes of bone pain and tiredness. In most cases, thinning of the bones is associated with spine and rib fractures. On the other hand, muscle weakness of the shoulders and hips occur in Cushing's syndrome.

Symptoms that are specific for men and women are also observed in cases of this disorder. In most cases, men may become impotent, or show decreased desire for sex. On the other hand, women with Cushing's syndrome experience interruptions in their menstrual cycles, a condition known as amenorrhea. They also have excessive hair growth on the thighs, chest, face, abdomen, and the neck (Newell-Price et al., 2006). In children, this disorder causes slow growth rate.

Other common symptoms that are associated with Cushing's syndrome include fatigue, headache, and mental changes, primarily anxiety or depression. Increased urination and thirst are also present in patients with this disorder (Newell-Price et al., 2006).

Genetic Basis for Cushing's Syndrome

Over the decades, there has been an intensive scientific inquiry into the genetic basis of Cushing's syndrome, primarily on the cause of excessive production of cortisol. However, most studies did not unravel the genetic mystery responsible for this phenomenon. It was only recently when genetic mutations were identified that facilitate the activation of Protein kinase A subunit. According to Beuschlein et al. (2014), somatic mutations in PRKACA gene are responsible for molecular changes in the production of cortisol by the adrenal cortex. Biologically, PRKACA gene is known to encode the cyclic AMP-dependent PKA subunit that is involved in the catalytic activation of cortisol-producing adenomas. Researchers in this study concluded that genetic alterations in somatic PRKACA are responsible for the production of excess cortisol in corticotropin-independent Cushing's syndrome cases (Beuschlein et al., 2014).

Diagnosis of Cushing's Syndrome

In practice, the diagnosis of Cushing's syndrome relies on a clinical review of the patient's physical examination, medical history and laboratory tests. Diagnosis focuses on determining the presence of excessive cortisol levels, combined with classic changes in body and facial appearance associated with Cushing's syndrome. Some of the recommended laboratory tests include 24-hour urinary cortisol test, low-dose dexamethasone suppression test and late-night salivary cortisol test. Others include MRI with gadolinium enhancement to identify tumors of the pituitary gland, and Petrosal sinus sampling. The latter is performed to determine the source of ACTH (Oldfield et al., 1991).

Treatment of Cushing's Syndrome

Microsurgical resection of pituitary adenomas responsible for secreting ACTH serves as the optimum treatment approach for this disorder. Surgery is usually followed by therapeutic treatment with drugs that inhibit cortisol production (Sharma & Nieman, 2011). Some of these drugs include Metyrapone (Metopirone), Mifepristone (Korlym), Ketoconazole (Nizoral), and Mitotane (Lysodren).

Conclusion

Conclusively, hormones play integral roles in maintaining homeostasis in the body. As such, disturbances in the regulatory hormone cascades results into clinical conditions as it is evidenced by Cushing's syndrome that develops due to disturbances of the HPA axis. In this condition, the body is exposed to excessive cortisol which is produced by tumors of the key endocrine glands, primarily the pituitary gland, adrenal gland, as well as, ectopic ACTH-producing tissues in the body. Overall, Cushing's syndrome is characterized by back pain, skin changes, muscles changes, and central obesity.

References

Beuschlein, F., Fassnacht, M., Assié, G., Calebiro, D., Stratakis, C.,... Osswald, A. (2014). Constitutive activation of PKA catalytic subunit in adrenal cushing's syndrome. *The New England Journal of Medicine, 370*, 1019-1028. doi: 10.1056/NEJMoa1310359

Hiller-Sturmhöfel, S., & Bartke, A. (1998). The endocrine system: an overview. *Alcohol Health & Research World, 22*(3), 153-164.

Newell-Price, J., Bertagna, X., Grossman, A., & Nieman, L. (2006). Cushing's syndrome. *The Lancet, 367*(9522), p1605–1617.

Oldfield, E., Doppman, J., Nieman, L., Chrousos, G., Miller, D., Katz, D.,... Cutler, G. (1991). Petrosal sinus sampling with and without corticotrophin-releasing hormone for the differential diagnosis of Cushing's syndrome. *The New England Journal of Medicine, 325*(13), 897-905. Retrieved from http://www.nejm.org/doi/pdf/10.1056/NEJM199109263251301

Sharma, S. T., & Nieman, L. K. (2011). Cushing's syndrome: all variants, detection, and treatment. *Endocrinol Metab Clin N Am., 40*, 379-391. PMID: 21565673

Vassiliadil, D., & Tsagarakis, S. (2007). Unusual causes of Cushing's syndrome. *Arquivos Brasileiros de Endocrinologia & Metabologia.* Retrieved from http://www.scielo.br/scielo.php?script=sci_arttext&pid=S0004-27302007000800010

YOUR KNOWLEDGE HAS VALUE

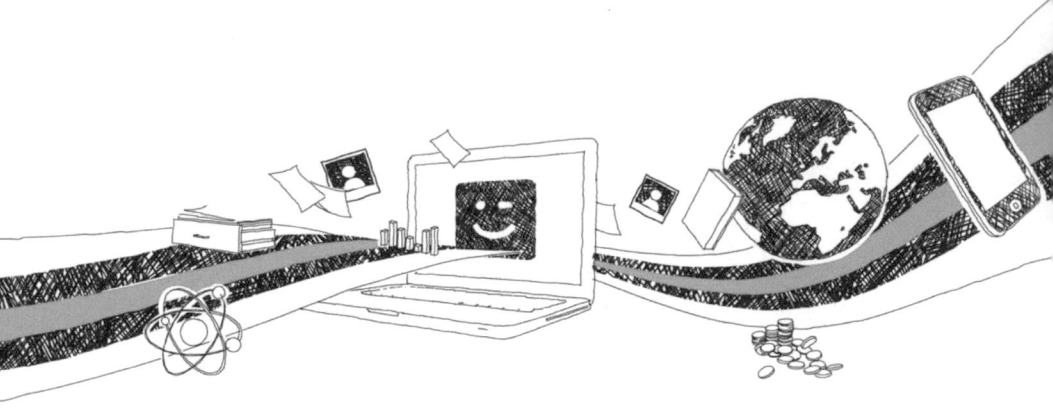

- We will publish your bachelor's and master's thesis, essays and papers

- Your own eBook and book - sold worldwide in all relevant shops

- Earn money with each sale

Upload your text at www.GRIN.com
and publish for free